Tapping for Weight Loss

The Beginner's Guide to Clearing Energy Blocks and Gaining Control of Your Weight Using the Emotional Freedom Technique

Lisa Townsend

Lisa Townsend

Table of Contents

Introduction

I want to thank you and congratulate you for purchasing, *"Tapping for Weight Loss - The Beginner's Guide to Clearing Energy Blocks and Gaining Control of Your Weight Using the Emotional Freedom Technique"*

Welcome to my beginner's guide to using the Emotional Freedom Technique (EFT or "tapping") for weight loss!

In this book, we will explore what tapping is, why it works, and how you can use it to remove the remove the emotional blocks that make losing weight an impossible dream.

Beginning with an overview of the Emotional Freedom Technique, this book breaks down the different parts of the technique and explains what they are, how to do them, and why they will help you lose those unwanted pounds. A detailed walk through of the standard tapping sequence and an in-depth explanation of each piece of the "basic recipe," position you not only to use the weight loss scripts provided here, but also to move forward and create your own tapping scripts that are unique to your situation.

I have included some ready-to-use tapping scripts that address common weight loss challenges like managing cravings and boosting self esteem. You can use these scripts to get started. Once you start removing those blocks, the knowledge provided here will help you identify other possible areas you may want to target to get the results you want.

After reading this guide, you will have a basic understanding of tapping away your unwanted weight you need to know to start tapping away your unwanted weight.

Lisa Townsend

What is the Emotional Freedom Technique?

Most people have heard of acupressure, acupuncture, and even Reiki, which are all forms of healing that use the human body's own energy field to help heal itself. The Emotional Freedom Technique (EFT) is another type of energy healing that uses a type of acupressure to help deal with the emotional issues that can stand in the way of making the healthy changes people need to make to improve their lives.

Developed in the 1990s by an acupuncturist named Gary Craig, EFT uses the widely accepted acupressure points in the body to release emotional energy blockages that keep us stuck in old, unhealthy patterns. The technique replaces the thin needles used in acupuncture with light taps of the fingers, which is why the technique is often called tapping.

EFT is a simple approach to removing the emotional and psychological blockages that keep us from achieving our goals. The beauty of the technique is that is it so simple, anyone can do it, and it is powerfully effective when done properly. Once you learn to perform the technique properly, you can do all the tapping yourself, at your own home, on your schedule.

Unfortunately, the simplicity that makes EFT such a great solution to this complex problem can create its own host of problems. People simply cannot believe that it can be as simple as it is. They change things to make it harder and more complex. While this might make them feel as though they are doing something more significant, the truth is that overcomplicating this simple process is more likely to decrease its effectiveness than it is to increase how well it works.

The Theory Behind EFT

The Emotional Freedom Technique is based on the principles espoused in Chinese medicine that the mind and body are connected through a field of energy.

This energy field contains energy channels called meridians that are part of the holistic healing system of the body. By tapping into the power of these meridians, energy healing techniques remove blockages which enable the body's own life-force to flow more freely. This life force, which is often called "qi" or "chi," needs to flow freely in order to initiate and sustain self-healing. According to this theory of dis-ease, illness and disease develop when blockages prevent the body from healing itself. When traditional Chinese techniques like acupuncture are used to remove those blockages, the flow of chi is restored, and the body is better able to prevent illness and heal dis-ease.

This is the theory on which EFT was built by Mr. Craig and his mentor Dr. Roger Callahan. They believed that the energy meridians used in acupuncture to prevent and treat physical ailments were also connected to our psychological and emotional health as well. Going on the understanding that physical health can be augmented using acupuncture, they believed that there had to be a way to access the emotional side of the energy meridians in order to remove blockages and take healing action. It was from this belief that EFT was born.

 Working from the hypothesis that energy meridians would provide a direct way access the emotional side of the energy meridians, Craig and Callahan developed EFT as a way to fully and permanently release the negative mental-emotional patterns responsible for the creation of our reality through the Law of Attraction. Basically, EFT provides a simple, practical, and highly effective way to change your energetic point of attraction. This can open the door to powerful self-change and an enormous capacity for self-healing. The basis of EFT can be explained with one sentence, coined The Discovery Statement by the founders of the technique.

"The cause of all negative emotions is simply a disruption in the body's energy system."

EFT restores our ability to self-heal by removing the blockage that is disrupting our energy system.

In acupuncture, the insertion of needles at specific points along the meridians is used to achieve these goals. In EFT, kinetic energy created by tapping the fingers against the body is used rather than the needles. When kinetic energy is added to these specific locations while focusing the mind on the problem that needs to be addressed and voicing the chosen affirmation, the emotional blockage that is holding you back is essentially short-circuited. This removes the blockage and realigns the balance between mind and body. This balance is the key to health, wellness, and longevity.

While many people remain skeptical of all energy-based healing techniques, these principles have been in use for more than 5,000 years as a part of Chinese medicine. The idea that there is a field of electromagnetic energy that flows throughout the body and that plays a significant role in health and healing is not a new concept. However, as medical practices begin to focus on a more holistic view of patient health even western medical practitioners are becoming more accepting of EFT and other energy alignment and healing techniques.

I can tell you from my own experience that EFT works. In fact, it is often more effective than other traditional or alternative methods at overcoming unhealthy emotional blockages and realigning or psychological energy for optimal health and healing. I have been using EFT exclusively with my patients for more than 10 years and am pleased to see that as others experience the success I have seen, acceptance of EFT as an effective therapeutic technique is spreading.

EFT can be used to prevent, treat, and address a wide range of issues including phobias, weight management problems, addiction, and even physical symptoms.

But How Does it Work?

There are two core elements involved in EFT. The first is tapping, which is the act of activating specific acupressure points. These are located at the end points of the energy meridians, and one activates them by tapping them with the fingertips. This inputs new kinetic energy into the meridian that helps to remove the blockage. The second is the verbal affirmation that is spoken that states the specific problem that needs to be addressed and an affirmation that will counteract that problem.

When these two elements combine, the emotional blockage related to the specified problem is removed and the balance of energy is adjusted. As more and more blockages are removed, the flow of chi improves, and the body's ability to heal itself is restored.

Tapping Basics

Tapping is one of the two core elements of EFT. Learning to do it properly is important in order for your EFT work to be successful. Successful tapping occurs when you can complete the sequence without having to think about it too much, so that your focus can remain on the process of release. For those new to tapping, it is often beneficial to practice the tapping part of the technique several times before adding the verbal component. This will allow you to become familiar enough with the sequence that you can focus on releasing the blockage.

The act of tapping creates kinetic energy, caused by the tapping of your fingertips that helps to release and remove the blockages along the energy meridians. This is why tapping in specific locations is important to the technique. The locations used in a tapping sequence are the end points of the energy meridians and are the same points used in other energy healing techniques.

While I have provided clear and complete instructions on how to use EFT here, there are countless video tutorials online that can be valuable resources to those new to the technique. When you are first starting out, it can be beneficial to watch someone else go through the tapping sequence a few times. This is especially true if you are a visual learner. Before you dive into the following chapters and start practicing your tapping technique, take a few minutes to look for a video online that resonates with you. The added benefit you will receive by watching someone else go through a tapping sequence or two will only make your efforts more successful in the end.

Locations

As I explained, the points used in the tapping sequence are the end points of the energy meridians. It is also important to know that there are also smaller meridian end points in the tip of each finger. So, when you use your fingertips to tap out the sequence you are getting an added benefit from these extra endpoints.

According to the original creators of EFT, only the index and middle fingers of one hand should be used to tap out the sequence. However, as the technique has evolved over the last two decades, other proponents of the technique have found that using all four fingers on both hands produces better results. For this reason, that is the method I recommend as I have seen the increased success of using these additional touch points. The key is to remember to use the fingertips rather than the pads of the fingers in order to get the extra boost from the meridian end points located there.

When tapping, the goal is to tap firmly, but your taps should never be hard enough to cause any pain. You can use one hand or both hands and even switch hands and sides during the sequence if that works best for you. Remember, the optimal way to run the tapping sequence is to do it in the way that requires the least amount of mental thought on your part. This ensures your focus and attention is on resolving the block rather than on where the next tap needs to be placed or with which hand.

Below is the conventional tapping sequence, laid out in order with a diagram of the specific location for the tap. Also included are the commonly used abbreviations you are likely to see in scripts you find from other sources for the locations. On each diagram, the black dot indicates where the tap should be placed.

The traditional sequence begins at the top of the head and flows down over the face to the collarbone before ending at the wrists.

1. Top of Head (TH)

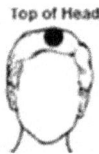

2. Eyebrow (EB)

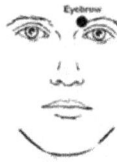

3. Side of Eye (SE)

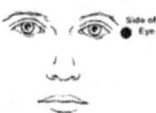

4. Under Eye (UE)

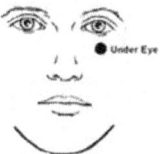

5. Under Nose (UN)

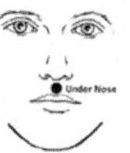

6.   Chin (Ch)

7.   Collarbone (CB)

8.   Under Arm (UA)

9.   Wrist (WR)

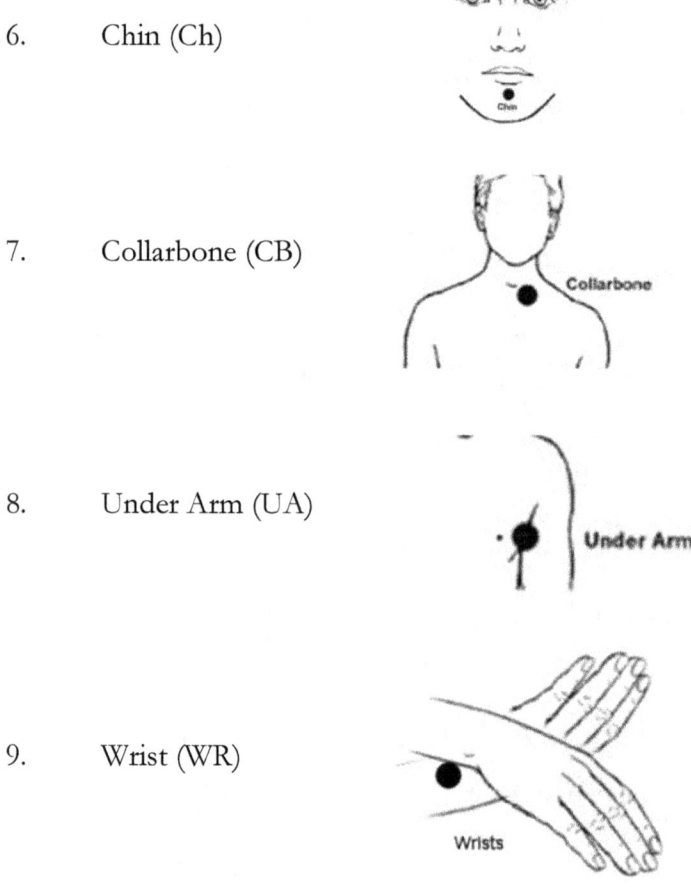

Note: The wrist tap is the only one not done with the finger tips. Instead, tap the insides of the wrists together.

Technique

In truth, the order in which you tap matters less than making sure you tap each of the locations in the sequence. Most people use this sequence because it is ordered in a way that makes it easy to remember each location. The reason the order doesn't matter is that EFT uses something called "the 100% overhaul concept". In essence, you are tapping all the energy meridians to make sure you get the right one.

Because EFT is a relatively new technique when compared to acupressure and acupuncture, we don't have a clear map of which meridian is tied to which kind of emotion or feeling. Without this map, we cannot do a more targeted tapping sequence because we don't have a clear picture as to which meridian needs to be involved in which kind of problem.

Additionally, when dealing with emotional and psychological issues, there is rarely a single source or factor involved. Because our emotions are so complex, it is possible that an issue like weight management could easily be blocked on certain meridians for one person and completely different meridians for another person. To account for this complexity, the tapping sequence covers all the bases to ensure any relevant blockages are removed.

Think of this tapping sequence as your total energetic overhaul. You are covering all the bases because tapping on a meridian that isn't blocked by the problem at hand won't hurt anything but missing one could jeopardize the whole process.

Affirmations

Now that you understand the mechanics of the tapping portion of the technique, it's time to move on to the second element, the verbal affirmation. Where the tapping allows you to tap into the energy flow of each meridian, the verbal affirmation is your tool to tune in to any blockages that are related to the problem you are trying to solve.

The affirmation statements are critical to the success of the technique, but you don't have to believe them in order for them to be effective. This is something many of my patients who are new to EFT are concerned about. As with any kind of affirmation, it is always better if you already believe it and can say it with emphasis, inflection, and passion. However, one of the main uses of affirmations is to change the way we think, which means we often don't believe them when we first begin using them.

Affirmations used for any purpose work better when they are said out loud, and the affirmation statements used in tapping are no exception. If you are around other people and feel uncomfortable, you can say them under your breath, but since they will still see you performing the tapping portion of the technique, you may be better off waiting until you are somewhere that you will feel comfortable doing both pieces openly and enthusiastically.

To understand how these affirmations help you tune in to any problems, we need to revisit the founder's Discovery Statement:

"The cause of all negative emotions is a disruption in the body's energy system."

What this essentially means is that when you tune into negative thoughts, they become negative emotions, and it is those emotions that cause the disruption in the body's energy field or system. Following that logic, directing your thoughts toward the problem you are trying to solve and focusing on the solution will have the opposite effect and remove the negative emotion and the disruption.

Here's what that could look like:

If you have spent years thinking about how fat you are or with your mind focused on how hard it is to lose weight, those negative thoughts are likely to have produced negative emotions related to your weight. You may feel fat, no matter what size you are. You might feel worthless or like a failure if you have tried and tried to lose weight to no avail. These negative emotions disrupt your body's energy system, making it even more difficult to lose weight by blocking the flow of chi and impeding the body's ability to self heal.

The first, best thing you can do is to tune into the problem so that the disruptions that are blocking your progress can be addressed.

Then, by changing that narrative and using affirmations that counteract that negativity, you can undo the damage to your energy system created by the initial negativity. Simply tuning in to the solution to the problem and letting go of the negative narrative makes it possible for the affirmation and the activation of the meridians to change the outcome you get. In this example, using tapping can make it possible to finally lose the extra weight you have been carrying around for years.

Why EFT for Weight Loss

One of the most powerful tools we have in the battle of the bulge is our own determination and perseverance. But past failures, rejections, and negative feedback about our weight can leave us with a lot of negativity towards ourselves and our ability to manage our weight. It is challenging to be determined and to keep pushing on when we feel dejected and worthless.

EFT helps correct that balance. It changes your narrative and eliminates the blocks caused by years of negative emotions regarding your weight. When you feel positive and hopeful, it is easier to do the things you need to do to accomplish your goals. When you remove all that negativity, you can learn to love the body you have, and this puts you firmly on track to get the body you want.

When you tap, the negative emotions and self-talk that are so corrosive that you keep them hidden in the back of your mind, come to the surface where they can be acknowledged and turned loose. This makes room for the positive thoughts and feelings that will support your journey to become who you want to be. When you clear out all that negative noise and get your body's energy system flowing, it is easier to understand what your body needs and what it doesn't.

Tapping helps with weight loss in several ways.

It can be used to overcome food cravings which are generally driven by emotions. Tapping helps release those emotions so that you aren't driven to eat that bag of chips or the package of cookies.

It is also used to correct and redirect the negative body image you carry around in your head and begin to love the body you are in. This is a critical piece of the tapping for weight loss program as it is often the biggest emotional hurdle that must be overcome to get back in touch with the body and focus on giving it what it needs to thrive.

EFT can also help with anxiety and self-sabotage, which can both impede weight loss efforts if they are not addressed.

Lisa Townsend

Recipe for Change

In EFT, the technique is often equated to a recipe. Just like a recipe, the ingredients and the order in which you do things are important. The "Basic Recipe," as I like to call it, makes it easy to do the right things in the right order every time, which is important if you want the technique to be as effective as possible. We talked about the two main ingredients, tapping and affirmations. Now let's look at how you put everything together to get results.

There are five steps in the Basic Recipe, broken down below to aid in understanding.

Choose a Problem

The very first thing you need to do is choose a specific problem that you want to address. When using tapping for weight loss, this problem can be a specific emotion you experience related to your weight, a traumatic event that is related to your weight, or a physical issue that is affecting your ability to lose weight. The most important thing about this step is choosing something that is very specific. If your problem statement is too general, the technique will not be as effective.

This doesn't mean you have to have the perfect problem statement before you can start. However, it does mean that you need something specific like "Fear that I will fail again if I try to lose weight on my own" rather than "Fear I will be fat forever."

You can find the problem statements that are applicable to you and your weight loss challenges by exploring your feelings about being overweight. Saying things like "I always

18

feel fat" and "I don't like what I see in the mirror" can bring up the triggering traumatic events, negative emotions, and basic beliefs that tied to your weight. As you encounter these, write them down and then review them to flesh out the specific problem statements you need to work through.

For example, if you say "I don't like what I see in the mirror," you might hear a voice in the back of your head that says, "Too bad, it's not like you are ever going to be able to lose any weight". That is one of the things that you believe about your weight, and it is one of the things that is holding you back. Taking that belief and transforming it into a problem statement could look something like, "Belief that it's not possible for me to be thinner and healthier." Once you understand the emotions, beliefs, and experiences that are getting in your way, you can take action to address them.

- Here are some examples of problem statements you might want to use in relation to weight loss.

- Fear that I won't lose those 20 pounds before my <u>insert event here</u>

- Fear that being overweight will give me diabetes

- Fear that if I lose the weight, I will only gain it back again

- Fear of interacting with the world without the fat to hide behind

- Fear that losing weight will change my relationships

- The time at the mall when that women asked me when my baby was due when I wasn't pregnant

- The time that guy I really liked said everything about me was perfect, I was just too fat for him to love

- Belief that it's not possible for me to be thinner and healthier

Rate the Intensity

The next step is to rate the intensity of the emotional response you are experiencing. That is done at the beginning and the end of every tapping session and again at the end of each tapping round within a session. When rating the intensity, use a scale from 1 to 10, where 1 is complete lack of distress and 10 is the most intense emotional distress you have ever experienced.

This is an important step because it helps you determine where you are and to see that you are making progress. It can also help you determine when you are done tapping for a specific problem. The goal of each tapping session is to bring that intensity level below a 2. Many times that cannot be accomplished with a single round of tapping.

When you are trying to choose from a list of potential problem statements, rank the intensity of each one. Then start with the one that has the highest intensity. If you have any that are already below a 2, you may need to dig deeper to see if there are any stronger emotional issues related to that problem. If not, you don't need to include it at this time.

As a reminder, this part of the process is about honestly rating your emotions right now. If you rate them how you want them to be, you are only cheating yourself out of changing them.

Create the Setup

The third step is to create the set-up, which is EFT-speak for the spoken phrase you will use to state the problem at the beginning of your tapping session. It will also influence the affirmation that will help you release the emotional energy tied to that problem. In this case, simple is best. The words are less important than their ability to focus your attention on clearing the block that your emotions are causing. If the words are too complicated, you won't be able to focus the way you need to.

It is also important to note that you do not have to change the words as you move through the session. Many online EFT scripts do this, and it can be effective for advanced practitioners. However, if you are struggling to remember which words you need to say at which point, you aren't focused on fixing the problem. Don't feel like you need to get fancy in order for this to be effective. In many cases, especially for those just starting out, simple will always be more effective.

Each set-up has three parts; the problem statement, the affirmation, and the reminder phrase.

The problem statement is one sentence that lays out the problem as specifically and concisely as possible. When crafting your problem statement, think of it as the directions you are giving yourself to find a specific recipe in your recipe box. If you say "I want to make a cake," it will be difficult to locate the specific recipe you want. Instead, you need to say something like "I want to make that German chocolate cake from my grandmother's recipe." This is very specific. That specificity makes it possible to find the exact recipe you want. Your problem statement needs to be specific enough that it allows you to access the actual emotion, event, or belief that is causing the blockage.

The affirmation is the phrase you will use to activate the healing mechanisms in your energy field that will deal with the problem from the problem statement. The most common format for EFT affirmations looks like this:

"Even though I (problem statement),
I deeply and profoundly love and accept myself."

While you can use affirmations that are not in this format, this one works well with EFT and helps keep things simple and easy. Just a reminder, you don't have to believe what you are saying when you say these affirmations. They still have power even if you don't believe them yet. As you move through the process of removing your emotional blocks, you will begin to see the truth in these affirmations and come to believe them yourself.

The reminder phrase is a small portion of the full set-up that you repeat as you perform the tapping sequence. The purpose of this phrase is to keep your attention focused on the problem you are trying to solve so that it remains activated in your energy field. This ensures you get the benefit of the tapping sequence.

The reminder phrase is repeated each time you tap to keep the problem activated for your subconscious. To see how this works, let's look at an example.

If your set-up is "Even though I have this fear that I won't lose these 20 pounds before my wedding, I deeply and profoundly love and accept myself." Your reminder phrase could be "won't lose 20 pounds" or "won't lose weight before wedding".

Tap the Sequence

The next step is to tap the sequence using a tapping script. A tapping script is simply step by step instructions for what to say and where to tap. It will use the abbreviations for each tapping location that were outlined above. As a refresher, the standard tapping sequence is:

1. Top of Head (TH)
2. Eyebrow (EB)
3. Side of Eye (SE)
4. Under Eye (UE)
5. Under Nose (UN)
6. Chin (Ch)
7. Collarbone (CB)
8. Under Arm (UA)
9. Wrist (WR)

There are many tapping scripts available online that are specific to weight loss, and I have included some in the next section. As you become more familiar with the process, you will be able to create your own scripts that are specific to your individual problems.

Rate the Intensity Again, and Repeat if Needed

The last step in each round of tapping is to rate the intensity again and record your ratings. This allows you to compare the intensity now to the intensity you were experiencing before completing a round of tapping. If your intensity is still over a 2, you need to perform another round of tapping. Repeat the process as many times as you need to in order to get that intensity rating below 2.

In subsequent rounds, you will need to make one simple change to the setup so that your subconscious knows you are working on clearing the remaining emotional blockage from the original issue rather than starting in on a new issue. The simple change is to add the word "still" to the set-up and the reminder phrase. For our example above, the set-up and reminder phrase for subsequent rounds of tapping would look like this:

"Even though I still have this fear that I won't lose these 20 pounds before my wedding, I deeply and profoundly love and accept myself." "Still won't lose 20 pounds."

Weight Loss Tapping Scripts

Now that you understand the process and the basic ingredients, it's time to put that know-how to work. Here are a few tapping scripts that address common problems people experience when trying to lose weight.

Problem #1 – Feeling Depressed About Weight

If you are feeling depressed or down about being overweight, you can use this script to help overcome those negative emotions and free up the energy they are blocking. Start by thinking about how being overweight makes you feel and doing the intensity rating for those emotions.

As you begin the tapping sequence, remember to speak out loud and with feeling in order to get the best result. The words you speak out loud are italicized.

Round #1

Say your set-up - Even *though I feel depressed about my weight, I deeply and profoundly love and accept myself.*

Say reminder phrase while tapping 5-7 times at each location

1. Top of Head (TH) – *depressed about weight*

2. Eyebrow (EB) – *depressed about weight*

3. Side of Eye (SE) – *depressed about weight*

4. Under Eye (UE) – *depressed about weight*

5. Under Nose (UN) – *depressed about weight*

6. Chin (Ch) – *depressed about weight*

7. Collarbone (CB) – *depressed about weight*

8. Under Arm (UA) – *depressed about weight*

9. Wrist (WR) – *depressed about weight*

Rate the intensity of the emotions. Compare with previous results. If needed, move on to additional rounds.

Round #2 and up

Say your set-up out loud - Even though I still feel depressed about my weight, I deeply and profoundly love and accept myself.

Say reminder phrase while tapping 5-7 times at each location

1. Top of Head (TH) – *still depressed about weight*

2. Eyebrow (EB) – *still depressed about weight*

3. Side of Eye (SE) – *still depressed about weight*

4. Under Eye (UE) – *still depressed about weight*

5. Under Nose (UN) – *still depressed about weight*

6. Chin (Ch) – *still depressed about weight*

7. Collarbone (CB) – *still depressed about weight*

8. Under Arm (UA) – *still depressed about weight*

9. Wrist (WR) – *still depressed about weight*

Rate the intensity of the emotions. Compare with previous results. If needed, move on to additional rounds. Once you reach a 2 or lower, you can end your session or move on to another set-up.

Problem #2 – Worried About Self Sabotage

One common problem many people who need to lose weight face is self-sabotage. The fear that we will derail our own progress this way can create energy disruptions that keep us from succeeding. You can use tapping to help address and release this fear. Start by thinking about the possibility of losing weight and then losing ground, of making progress, only to wind up back where you started. Capture the emotions that come up with these thoughts and do the intensity rating for those emotions.

This script is a little different as it involves two rounds with two different set-ups and uses slightly different reminder phrases at each tapping location, rather than repeating the same reminder phrase each time.

Round #1

Say your set-up - Even though I have sabotaged myself in the past, and I will certainly sabotage myself in the future, I deeply and profoundly love and accept myself.

Say reminder phrase while tapping 5-7 times at each location

1.   Top of Head (TH) – *I know I will sabotage myself in the future.*

2.   Eyebrow (EB) – *I acknowledge that I have sabotaged myself in the past.*

3.   Side of Eye (SE) – *Being self sabotaging is inevitable.*

4.   Under Eye (UE) – *I have always sabotaged my weight loss efforts in the past.*

5.   Under Nose (UN) – *I know I will sabotage my weight loss efforts in the future.*

6.   Chin (Ch) – *I know I will undo any good that I have done by sabotaging myself.*

7.   Collarbone (CB) – *I am an expert at sabotaging my weight loss goals.*

8.   Under Arm (UA) – *I will always sabotage my weight loss goals.*

9.   Wrist (WR) – *I will never lose weight because I sabotage myself.*

Wait to rate the intensity until after the second round.

Round #2

Say your set-up - Even though I am an expert at sabotaging myself, and it is something I always do, I deeply and profoundly love and accept myself.

Say reminder phrase while tapping 5-7 times at each location

1. Top of Head (TH) – *I will definitely sabotage myself in the future.*

2. Eyebrow (EB) – *But maybe this time I won't.*

3. Side of Eye (SE) – *I can choose to change my behavior.*

4. Under Eye (UE) – *I am a different person than I was every other time.*

5. Under Nose (UN) – *I know more than I did before, I have better skills and tools.*

6. Chin (Ch) – *I can choose to be different this time.*

7. Collarbone (CB) – *I can create the future I want.*

8. Under Arm (UA) – *I can lose weight without sabotaging myself.*

9. Wrist (WR) – *I can let go of my fear of self-sabotage.*

Rate the intensity of the emotions. Compare with previous results. If needed, move on to additional rounds. If you need to do additional rounds, make sure you add "still" to the set-ups and reminder phrases. Once you reach a 2 or lower, you can end your session or move on to another set-up.

Problem #3 – Feeling Like I Will Never Lose This Weight

If you feel like losing weight is impossible and that you will never be able to lose the weight, you can use this script to help overcome those negative emotions and free up the energy they are blocking. This script is more complicated than the others included here and provides a good example of how you can customize your tapping scripts once you become more familiar with the process. Just remember, scripts do not have to have this level of complexity to be effective.

Start off by thinking about why you feel like you will never lose weight and doing the intensity rating for those emotions.

As you begin the tapping sequence, remember to speak out loud and with feeling in order to get the best result. The words you speak out loud are italicized.

Round #1

Set-up - Even though I feel like I will never lose this extra weight, I choose to feel positive and allow myself to release this extra weight now.

Say reminder phrase while tapping 5-7 times at each location

1. Top of Head (TH) – *I don't believe I will ever lose weight*

2. Eyebrow (EB) – *I'm convinced I will always be fat.*

3. Side of Eye (SE) – *I don't believe I will lose this extra weight.*

4.   Under Eye (UE) – *I must want to be fat, there must be something in it for me.*

5.   Under Nose (UN) – *Something inside of me thinks that being fat is better.*

6.   Chin (Ch) – *I may think being fat keeps people at a distance.*

7.   Collarbone (CB) – *I may believe that if people stay away I can't get hurt.*

8.   Under Arm (UA) – *I may be anxious about the attention being thin would bring.*

9.   Wrist (WR) – *Yes, being fat feels more comfortable, and I would rather be comfortable than risk change.*

Wait to gauge your intensity until the end of the session.

Round #2

Skip the set-up in this round.

Say reminder phrase while tapping 5-7 times at each location

1. Top of Head (TH) – *What if I could let go of these negative feelings about my weight.*

2. Eyebrow (EB) – *What if I could feel positive about being thin and healthy.*

3. Side of Eye (SE) – *What if losing the extra weight made me feel better.*

4. Under Eye (UE) – *What if I could let go of the extra weight and the fear of change.*

5. Under Nose (UN) – *What if I could let losing weight be a positive change.*

6. Chin (Ch) – *What if I gave myself permission to start losing weight now.*

7. Collarbone (CB) – *What if I could feel comfortable about having a thinner body.*

8. Under Arm (UA) – *What if I could let go of my anxiety about getting attention if I was thin.*

9. Wrist (WR) – *What if I could lose the extra weight and keep it off forever.*

Wait to gauge your intensity until the end of the session.

Round #3

Skip the set-up in this round.

Say reminder phrase while tapping 5-7 times at each location

1.   Top of Head (TH) – *I am ready to choose to let go of these feelings about my weight.*

2.   Eyebrow (EB) – *I am ready to choose to feel positive about being thin and healthy.*

3.   Side of Eye (SE) – *I am ready to choose to believe that losing the extra weight will make me feel better.*

4.   Under Eye (UE) – *I am ready to choose to let go of the extra weight and the fear of change.*

5.   Under Nose (UN) – *I am ready to choose to let losing weight be a positive change.*

6.   Chin (Ch) – *I am ready to choose to give myself permission to start losing weight now.*

7.   Collarbone (CB) – *I am ready to choose to feel comfortable about having a thinner body.*

8.   Under Arm (UA) – *I am ready to choose to let go of my anxiety about getting attention if I am thin.*

9.   Wrist (WR) – *I am ready to choose to lose the extra weight and keep it off forever.*

Wait to gauge your intensity until the end of the session.

Round #4

Skip the set-up in this round.

Say reminder phrase while tapping 5-7 times at each location

1. Top of Head (TH) — *I choose to be grateful for the body I have right now.*

2. Eyebrow (EB) — *I choose to be grateful for all the weight I can safely lose now.*

3. Side of Eye (SE) — *I am grateful that I can release all the negative feelings I have about my weight.*

4. Under Eye (UE) — *I am grateful that I can choose to push past fear and have the body I deserve to have.*

5. Under Nose (UN) — *I am grateful that I always feel fantastic when I look in the mirror.*

6. Chin (Ch) — *I am grateful that I can picture myself without the extra weight in a positive way.*

7. Collarbone (CB) — *I grateful for the body I have right now and for the body I am working to have in the future.*

8. Under Arm (UA) — *I am grateful that I have the strength to make the choices I need to make to have a new life.*

9. Wrist (WR) — *I am grateful that I can allow myself to feel positive about my body.*

Rate your intensity level. If you have emotions that are still above a 2, repeat the session.

Conclusion

Throughout this book, it has been my intention to lay out a clear path to creating a framework for you to use EFT to help you achieve your weight loss goals. I believe you should have a firm foundation from the information here to begin using EFT and tapping to help you achieve your goals.

As you move forward and begin putting the information you learned into practice, I urge you to let go of any attempts to control the technique with your mind. Remember, you will make the most progress when you let go and trust the process to work. Put your faith in your own subconscious and let it get to the work of self-healing. The more you trust yourself to handle this kind of healing, the easier it will be for the tapping to do its work.

It's been my privilege to guide you at this stage in your journey, and I congratulate you on taking the next step towards achieving your goal weight. I know that with perseverance and consistency these techniques will support you in making the life changes you want to make.

Wishing you peace, joy, and fulfillment on your journey to a bigger and brighter life.

Namaste!

Lisa Townsend

Check out some of Lisa's other books!!

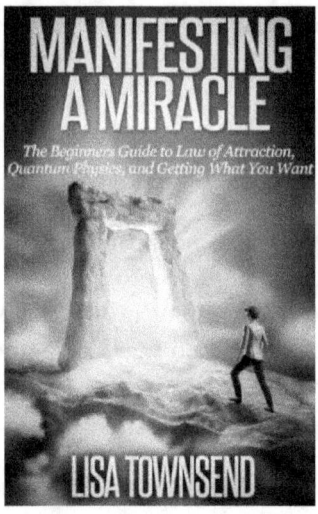

http://www.amazon.com/dp/B00IXCUGWE

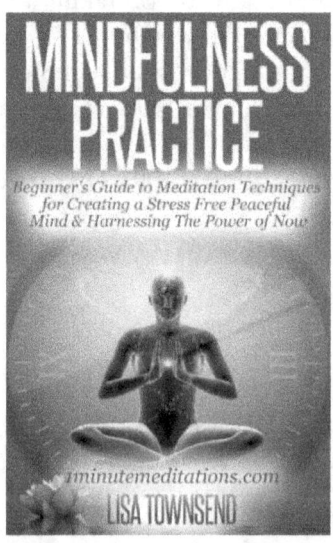

http://www.amazon.com/dp/B00IX71JQQ

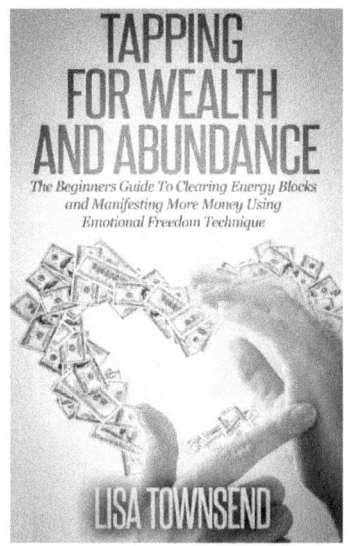

http://www.amazon.com/dp/B00K37EXW6

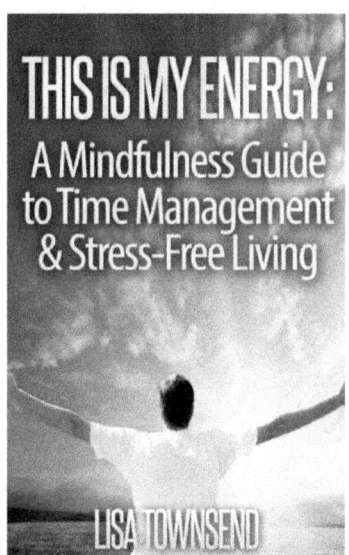

http://www.amazon.com/dp/B00K1N9Q56